Public Health and Soft Power

The Republic of Korea's Initial COVID-19 Response and Its Implications for Health Diplomacy

JENNIFER BOUEY, LYNN HU, SOHAELA AMIRI, RAFIQ DOSSANI

Prepared for the Korea Foundation

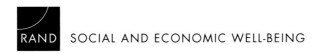

RAND SOCIAL AND ECONOMIC WELL-BEING

For more information on this publication, visit **www.rand.org/t/RRA1415-1**.

About RAND

The RAND Corporation is a research organization that develops solutions to public policy challenges to help make communities throughout the world safer and more secure, healthier and more prosperous. RAND is nonprofit, nonpartisan, and committed to the public interest. To learn more about RAND, visit www.rand.org.

Research Integrity

Our mission to help improve policy and decisionmaking through research and analysis is enabled through our core values of quality and objectivity and our unwavering commitment to the highest level of integrity and ethical behavior. To help ensure our research and analysis are rigorous, objective, and nonpartisan, we subject our research publications to a robust and exacting quality-assurance process; avoid both the appearance and reality of financial and other conflicts of interest through staff training, project screening, and a policy of mandatory disclosure; and pursue transparency in our research engagements through our commitment to the open publication of our research findings and recommendations, disclosure of the source of funding of published research, and policies to ensure intellectual independence. For more information, visit www.rand.org/about/research-integrity.

RAND's publications do not necessarily reflect the opinions of its research clients and sponsors.

Published by the RAND Corporation, Santa Monica, Calif.
© 2022 RAND Corporation
RAND® is a registered trademark.

Library of Congress Cataloging-in-Publication Data is available for this publication.
ISBN: 978-1-9774-1003-0

Cover: Photo by Thomas Maresca/UPI/ Alamy Stock Photo.

Limited Print and Electronic Distribution Rights

About This Report

During the early days of the coronavirus disease 2019 (COVID-19) pandemic in 2020, the Republic of Korea (ROK) had one of the highest success rates in adopting effective nonpharmaceutical interventions to rapidly contain the virus without a national lockdown. The ROK government's proactive strategy for nonpharmaceutical intervention adoption has received global attention for its success. The objective of the report is to understand the advantage and limitations of health diplomacy and identify the possible strategies for the ROK to turn its COVID-19 response success into a successful soft power asset for health diplomacy in the future. The report is based on a comprehensive literature review of ROK's COVID-19 pandemic responses in the first six months of 2020 and on pandemic preparedness, soft power, and health diplomacy. We also conducted in-depth interviews with Asian country experts in public health and international relationship for additional insights and guidance on the analysis. The Korea Foundation provided the funding for the project from 2021 to 2022. The research will be of value to policymakers who are interested in the subject of strengthening soft power through health diplomacy.

Community Health and Environmental Policy Program

RAND Social and Economic Well-Being is a division of the RAND Corporation that seeks to actively improve the health and social and economic well-being of populations and communities throughout the world. This research was conducted in the Community Health and Environmental Policy Program within RAND Social and Economic Well-Being. The program focuses on such topics as infrastructure, science and technology, community design, community health promotion, migration and population dynamics, transportation, energy, and climate and the environment, as well as other policy concerns that are influenced by the natural and built environment, technology, and community organizations and institutions that affect well-being. For more information, email chep@rand.org.

Acknowledgments

We would like to thank the RAND Center for Asia Pacific Policy for its support in grant proposal review and interview referral support during the project, and to the interviewees, all of whom gave generously of their time and knowledge to convey their understanding of this difficult topic. Finally, we thank the reviewers of this report, Chris Nelson and Seow Ting Lee, for their time, expertise, and diligence.

Summary

Issue

In 2020, during the early days of the coronavirus disease 2019 (COVID-19) pandemic, nations around the world—hampered by the lack of a basic understanding of the virus, including its mode of transmission and the risk factors for infection and disease—had to rely on nonpharmaceutical interventions, including physical barriers, social distancing, symptom screening, contract tracing, and case isolation. During this period, the Republic of Korea (ROK) had one of the highest success rates in adopting effective nonpharmaceutical interventions to contain the virus, rapidly achieving virus containment and suffering very low mortality without a national lockdown. The ROK government's proactive "three T" strategy for nonpharmaceutical intervention adoption—testing, tracing, and treatment triage—has received global attention for its success. This report considers whether this strategy has other potential benefits. In particular, we ask whether and how the ROK can turn its COVID-19 control success into a successful "soft power asset" for health diplomacy.

Soft power is the ability to influence others to obtain desired outcomes through attraction rather than coercion or payment. Without relying on hard power from military strength and economic size, a country can apply its soft power to attract collaborations, shape the international agenda, and reduce conflicts. In this report, we identify the characteristics of the ROK government's initial response to COVID-19 and assess how these characteristics might be translated into soft power assets despite the limitations and risks of health diplomacy; and make recommendations to support the ROK in building and strengthening its soft power globally.

Research Approach

We carried out a comprehensive literature review of the ROK's control strategies in the early stages of the COVID-19 pandemic, as documented in government and think tank white papers, scientific literature, and news reports. We also examined the foundations for ROK's public health actions by assessing ROK's pandemic response readiness using the World Health Organization's (WHO's) Joint External Evaluation reports and a survey of scientific literature on the foundations of the preparedness and on soft power. We consulted global health experts, government officials, and practitioners in several Asian countries, including the ROK, in multiple waves to obtain guidance and feedback on our analysis and policy recommendations.

Key Findings

Soft Power Can Increase a Country's Global Influence but Also Involves Risk

A nation's soft power assets range from its system of governance to its resources, such as capital, skilled labor, access to technology, information, partnerships, and networks. Soft power can be built through collaboration between government, academic, and commercial institutions as an alternative to armed conflict or economic negotiation. Health diplomacy can enhance soft power through building global health governance even during conflicts between countries. Many countries also apply health diplomacy to build long-term soft power for security purpose.

While soft power and health diplomacy can be beneficial, the use of soft power can sometimes encounter barriers and limitations and can have unintended consequences. We considered four types of limitations and risks associated with soft power assets, including (1) collateral damage when the values and practices of a soft power asset appear to be at odds with a target country's values and norms; (2) misunderstandings and negative perceptions triggered by cultural and language barriers; (3) fear and resistance triggered when soft power resources are awkwardly applied and, thus, perceived as a form of coercion and manipulation; and (4) inability to sustain soft power assets, which are often outside government control.

The ROK's Initial COVID-19 Success Provides a Solid Foundation for Health Diplomacy

We identified six main features of the ROK's success in containing COVID-19 during the pandemic, which could be the source of soft power through public health diplomacy:

1. *A sensitive pandemic alert system and pandemic preparation.* Early alerts allowed the ROK government to enhance early case screening at borders and develop diagnostic tools, establish response plans, and secure human resources for the epidemic control even before the country's first outbreak.
2. *A centralized hierarchical response system to coordinate pandemic resource allocation and risk communication.* As soon as pandemic response protocols were activated, the ROK prime minister, together with two other ministers, established the Central Disaster and Safety Countermeasure Headquarters and Control Tower. This headquarters was instrumental in mobilizing medical resources, building an emergency public-private partnership for supplies and production, and communicating with the public.
3. *COVID-19 national testing strategy.* The early and rapid expansion of COVID-19 testing was built on two critical developments in the ROK, which were prompted by its 2015 experience with Middle East respiratory syndrome (MERS): (1) In 2017, the ROK made a U.S. $25-million investment in infectious disease diagnostic technology, which established a key public and private partnership for diagnostic testing, and (2) the ROK established an agency-led emergency use authorization program to fast track test kits during pandemics.
4. *Stringent infection tracing and containment strategies.* In the first year of the pandemic, the ROK established stringent contact tracing and containment strategies, implementing a strict quarantine and isolation strategy.

5. *Information and communication technology applications.* Various of these technologies supported the contact tracing and containment strategy, including a self-quarantine safety application and an epidemiological investigation support system.
6. *A two-track COVID-19 hospital triage system.* The ROK redesigned health service provision at the national level for COVID-19. A national-level coordination center managed the flow of COVID-19 patients to hospitals or, if needed, to other provinces, while patients with non-COVID-19 conditions were sent to what were called system *safety guaranteed hospitals.*

The ROK possesses several attributes that helped the country manage the initial response to the COVID-19 pandemic well, including social homogeneity, a superb health care system, and technology resources, along with significant economic power and a governing style that includes strict penalties for policy violations. Other key components of the early success include the transparent and effective government-public communications the nation established after the MERS outbreaks in 2015 and a high level of compliance with public health protocols among the ROK public. The ROK's pandemic response scored well on the WHO's Joint External Evaluation indicators pre–COVID-19, especially in the domains of national coordination and health finance; testing, surveillance, and contact tracing; and supplies and workforce management.

The ROK Has the Potential to Demonstrate Soft Power and Avoid Risks

The ROK can leverage its success with the initial response to COVID-19 to demonstrate soft power assets that span multiple domains identified by a theory-based soft power index *Soft Power 30,* including (1) digital resources and technological advancement, (2) private enterprise resources, (3) education and labor market resources, (4) cultural resources, (5) engagement activities, and (6) government capacity.

When attempting to apply these assets, however, the ROK should develop a proactive strategy to address areas of limitations and potential risks. For example, the ROK's technological capabilities for performing large-scale testing have been important for boosting the nation's image; however, applying this asset might also raise concerns about privacy and other legal and political issues related to the government's use of individuals' private data to facilitate digital contact tracing. Such concerns might be addressed by emphasizing the ROK's role as a democratic country that has a pandemic infectious disease law allowing the government to use private data in this way. It is important to acknowledge and address such risks when designing strategies for using soft power assets in health diplomacy.

Finally, such strategies as building decentralized channels for engagement, utilizing ROK embassies for linguistic and cultural guidance, and developing a sustainable long-term financial plan for science diplomacy initiatives can also help the ROK avoid common limitations and risks associated with health diplomacy.

Policy Recommendations

The ROK has an opportunity to promote its image and status in the global health and foreign policy hierarchy. Our research offers some recommendations to support the ROK in building and strengthening its soft power globally.

- **Build ROK soft power by leveraging the nation's advanced biomedical and digital technology, as in the early development and production of COVID-19 testing.** Such a strategy should emphasize that the digital technology used in disease tracking and quarantine monitoring was based on citizens' agreement on privacy rights unique to a pandemic era and anchored in the infectious disease law. To minimize the perception of market coercion, manufacturing hubs and alliances should be open to assisting other countries' economies and supporting technology transfer.

- **Build the ROK's soft power through public health science diplomacy.** ROK public health agencies and universities that conducted training during the pandemic can be modeled as regional pandemic response training centers, and public health agencies can support ROK universities and develop peer-to-peer global research and teaching networks and public health degree programs. To build education capacity, it will be necessary to offer educational resources in many languages, promote cultural openness, and build a long-term financial plan.

- **Build the ROK's soft power through civil society and governmental exchange programs.** The ROK's success in the COVID-19 response illustrates that the democratic system does not necessarily cause disputes over public health mandates. Decentralized civil organization exchange programs, and inviting government delegations to visit COVID-19 pandemic response projects can aid in the promotion of global networks, dialogues, and health diplomacy.

- **Build the ROK's soft power through engagement with international multilateral agencies and humanitarian aid.** COVID-19 has strengthened the nation's capabilities in health diplomacy, including engagement with multilateral global health organizations (e.g., WHO Access to COVID-19 Tools Accelerator, Gavi, the Vaccine Alliance), and has strengthened alliances with Asia Pacific countries (via the Association of Southeast Asian Nations). To maintain such momentum, the ROK will need to sustain the funding and align the interests and priorities of different government ministries. The ROK can also leverage its embassies' guidance and resources to help health care professional training and humanitarian aid projects with language and culture adaptations in international settings.

Contents

Figures and Tables

Figures

Tables

Chapter 1. Introduction

A modern global health and humanitarian disaster, the coronavirus disease 2019 (COVID-19) pandemic, presented unprecedented challenges in multiple stages: the initial encounters, the development of medical interventions, and the implementation of the interventions. In comparison with other high-income nations, the Republic of Korea (ROK) has successfully maintained its low COVID-19 death rate and a thriving economy.[1] Such success is highly dependent on the nation's remarkable initial response to the pandemic, which will be the focus of this report. At the time the pandemic broke out, public health responses to it were hampered by the lack of a basic understanding of the virus's epidemiologic characteristics, including its mode of transmission and risk factors for infection and disease. Without a vaccine and effective treatment or accurate testing tools, countries had to rely on nonpharmaceutical interventions, including physical barriers, social distancing, known symptom screening, contract tracing, and case isolation. As of February 2020, the ROK had the second-highest number of cases in the world, following China. However, an effective response rapidly contained the virus, and the country suffered very low mortality without a national lockdown (Oh et al., 2020; Choi et al., 2020) and maintained a low incidence rate of COVID-19 until the fall of 2020, when the pandemic entered a new stage, with vaccines in the last stages of clinical trials and new variants of the virus spreading. The ROK government's proactive "three T" strategy for nonpharmaceutical intervention adoption—testing, tracing, and treatment triage—has received global attention for its success (Park et al., 2020; Rokni and Park, 2020; Schaller, 2020).

In the same years of the COVID-19 pandemic, global geopolitics and power competitions in the Asia-Pacific entered a new era. *Soft power* refers to a country's ability to attract and influence other nations and to build enduring international partnerships. According to soft power experts, countries that had successful pandemic responses are likely to see their soft power rise (McClory, 2021). At the same time, there was also strong pushback against some "mask" or "vaccine" diplomacy (Verma, 2020). Thus, a key issue for the ROK is whether its success in COVID-19 can be turned into a soft power asset and can serve as a springboard to enhance the nation's global presence in pandemic preparedness.

Research Goal and Research Questions

The goal of this research was to provide strategies and policy recommendations on how to translate the successful initial response to COVID-19 into soft power assets through health

---

[1] The cumulative COVID-19 death rate as of June 16, 2022, was 477 per million in the ROK compared to an average 2,002 per million in high-income countries, according to "Coronavirus Pandemic (COVID-19)," undated.

1

diplomacy safely and realistically in the post–COVID-19 world. Traditional public health papers seldom tap into theories of soft power, and national security studies do not dive deeply into public health delivery. Although some studies have examined the ROK's national branding post–COVID-19 (Lee and Kim, 2021; Dewi and Auliyah, 2022; Hidayatullah, 2021), we further focused specifically on health diplomacy and soft power in this project. In this report, we seek to answer the following questions:

- What is soft power, and what advantages, limitations, and risks are associated with building soft power from health diplomacy?
- What were the characteristics of the ROK government's successful initial COVID-19 response? What was the foundation of the ROK's COVID-19 response?
- Can these pandemic response and foundation characteristics be turned into soft power assets for ROK? When doing so, what limitations should be kept in mind and what common risks associated with health diplomacy should be avoided?

Organization of This Report

Chapter 2 focuses on soft power and health diplomacy and the advantages and risks associated with the use of health diplomacy. Chapter 3 examines the successful features of the ROK's COVID-19 response and discusses their implications for the potential use of soft power assets. Chapter 4 expands on the soft power asset analysis by examining the cultural and health system foundations of the response. Chapter 5 provides policy recommendations.

Our approach included a comprehensive literature review of the response in the ROK and a few other Asian countries, an analysis of soft power assets based on the six-domain framework of SP30, and the incorporation of in-country subject experts' guidance and feedback. The appendix describes our research methodology in detail.

Chapter 2. Soft Power and Health Diplomacy Post–COVID-19

Soft Power and Its Measurement

Developing and delivering effective foreign policy in today's ever-more globalized and contested world is challenging. More powerful interests, more platforms, and more actors are vying for global influence. Countries with limited hard power rooted in military strength and economic weight can still win political clout and shape regional and international agendas when they invest in soft power (Nye, 2004). Nye defines *soft power* as "the ability to obtain the preferred outcomes one wants by attraction rather than coercion or payment" (Nye, 2017). A state's soft power assets lie primarily in its culture, values, and foreign policies (Nye, 2004). More recently, others have argued that a nation's soft power assets range from its system of governance to its resources, such as capital, skilled labor, access to technology, information, partnerships, and networks (Amiri, 2022). While soft power is rarely sufficient on its own to resolve real-world situations, it can be a force multiplier in the world of politics. With the unpredictable geopolitics surrounding great power competitions in the post–COVID-19 era, stronger soft power can improve the ROK's ability to build regional and global alliances that produce long-term security benefits for the ROK and its citizens. In doing so, health diplomacy can also improve regional and global disease controls and reduce catastrophic risks to the ROK.

Multiple indexes exist that measure a country's soft power. We examined three of these: the Brand Finance's global soft power index (Brand Finance, undated), Monocle's soft power survey index (Monocle, 2017), and Portland's Soft Power 30 (SP30). We chose SP30 as the primary index because it has the most-comprehensive quantitative measurements of the three and because its theoretical base has the closest alliance with the Nye's soft power concept. SP30 is built on Joseph Nye's theory of soft power and includes more than 75 metrics and seven categories of annual international polling data from 25 countries of major geopolitical regions.

Compared with the Brand Finance index, which focuses primarily on financial branding, SP30 provides a comprehensive assessment of a country's influence in six subdomains (digital, enterprise, education, culture, engagement, and government). Compared with Monocle's five-domain soft power index, SP30 added digital media and combines analysis of standard databases and a multicountry polling score. The global polling focuses on subjective impressions of foreign policy, friendliness, culture, technology products, cuisine, livability, and luxury goods. While the index is far from perfect, it is by far one of the most-comprehensive tools to measure countries' soft power resources (McClory, 2015; McClory, 2019).

Health Diplomacy as a Soft Power Tool

Given our report's focus on COVID-19 and global health assistance policy, we will primarily look into the association between soft power and health diplomacy in this report. The concept of *medical diplomacy* as means of improving international relations was first introduced in 1978 by Peter Bourne, when he was a special presidential assistant in the Carter administration (Bourne, 1978). While traditional diplomacy focuses on economics and security, health diplomacy is *concerned with health and humanitarian interests.* (Watkins, 2020). Rebecca Katz has identified three types of health diplomacy: core diplomacy (e.g., treaties among countries), multistakeholder diplomacy (e.g., international partnerships), and informal diplomacy (e.g., government staff in the field interact with the public and nongovernmental organizations) (Katz et al., 2011).

Health diplomacy can be used to support global health governance and improve relationships between countries through health policies and initiatives that serve to counterbalance conflicts between the countries (Katz et al., 2011; Kickbusch and Liu, 2022). Historical examples include the successful development and administration of a rabies vaccine by the Pasteur Institute's network of laboratories in Indochina and North Africa during colonial wars (1892–1897) and the collaboration between the United States and the Soviet Union at the peak of the Cold War (1956–1959) to develop polio and smallpox vaccines (Hotez, 2014).

Not only can successful health diplomacy improve global health during conflicts, it can also improve a country's soft power and enhance its ability to build public goods and, in turn, to protect its own citizens. For decades, the United States has demonstrated its ample resources in biotechnology and public health through its investments in global institutions and has served as the top donor and key technical advisor for multilateral international organizations. The Global Health Initiative—a signature initiative formed during the Obama administration—was launched in 2009 to tie together U.S. global health programs, such as the President's Plan for AIDS Relief and the President's Malaria Initiative, and programs on maternal and children's health, family planning, neglected tropical diseases, and other critical health areas (Clinton, 2010). Hillary Clinton, as Secretary of State in the Obama administration, famously stated that the United States should invest in global health to "strengthen fragile and failing states, to promote social and economic progress, and to protect U.S. security" (Global Health Europe, 2010).

Western democratic allies are not the only nations that have recognized and implemented health diplomacy as a soft power tool to gain friends and influence. Cuba established Cuban medical internationalism in 1959 to provide direct health care and health care professional training. More than 40,000 personnel have deployed to nearly 100 countries since then, and the largest global medical school—Escuela Latinoamericana de Medicina—has enrolled more than 8,000 students from the developing world (Feinsilver, 2008). China has a long history of sending medical missions to third-world countries to build solidarity with them and to secure its political clout and standing on international platforms (Bouey, 2019; Bouey, 2020). Egypt recently applied health diplomacy by sending medical convoys for Nile Basin countries, donating medical supplies to China and African countries, and building health services facilities in Lebanon and other countries (Elsayed, 2020). Commenting on the value of health diplomacy, an African global health scholar recently noted that soft power built through health diplomacy will "win over the hearts and minds of citizens, as well as can help set the international health agenda" (Watkins, 2020).

Health Diplomacy's Limitations and Risks

While health diplomacy can be beneficial for building soft power, there are limits to what it can achieve. First, Nye noted that government policies at home and abroad are a potential source of soft power. Domestic health policies that appear in a different cultural norm to be hypocritical or to infringe on rights can undermine the country's soft power. Second, overseas health diplomacy implementations also often rely on nongovernment entities—individuals, organizations, and companies—outside the government's direct control. Third, soft power assets can also take a long time to show results in building soft power. (Nye, 2019). Even with extensive soft power assets and good intentions, a government's ability to sustain soft power can be limited.

In addition to the limitations, we should also be aware of the risks—the unintended backlash or unpredictable returns—associated with health diplomacy. Take the polio eradication effort in Afghanistan, for example. The U.S. implementation ran into various obstacles, including security issues, difficulties in maintaining a cold supply chain for vaccines, challenges in setting up active and sentinel surveillance, the emergence of false beliefs about vaccines, and distrust of health care workers. These problems not only resulted in the continued persistence of polio in Afghanistan but also left many locals with the perception that the U.S. health diplomacy effort was intended as coercion (Shakeel et al., 2019). Similarly, some countries lauded China's medical team, vaccine, and mask diplomacy efforts during COVID-19 (e.g., Serbia, Italy, Spain, and Netherland), but the efforts caused controversy in others (e.g., Turkey, because of negative perceptions of China's handling of COVID-19 and China's delayed delivery of vaccines it had promised) (Demir, 2021). Beijing's soft power projection also intensified the rivalry between the United States and China (Gauttam, Singh, and Kaur, 2020).

Thus, before engaging in health diplomacy activities, a country would do well to make a careful evaluation of the potential limitations and risks of each soft power asset. Hill and Beadle (2014) summarized four types of limitations and risks associated with soft power assets. First, collateral damage can arise when the values and practices of a soft power asset are celebrated at home but appear to be at odds with a recipient country's values and norms. For example, it is considered acceptable for the government to use private credit card information to trace virus spread in the ROK, but concerns about the privacy of citizens' data arose in other countries when such practices were introduced to other countries. Second, cultural and language barriers can often trigger misunderstandings and negative perceptions. One example concerns the negative sentiments provoked by foreign health care professionals who are oblivious to the depth of poverty or limits of medical facilities in the regions they visited (Martiniuk et al., 2012). Third, as noted above, fear and resistance can be triggered if soft resources are awkwardly applied and, thus, perceived as a form of coercion and manipulation. For example, China's mask diplomacy backfired when officials asked recipient countries to openly express gratitude toward China (Jacinto, 2020). Finally, the sustainability of soft power assets is often in question because they can be outside the government's budget (unlike military power). Thus, sustainability requires multisector collaboration and intense (e.g., digital platform) and/or long-term (e.g., culture, education) investment.

To minimize these limitations and risks, we will apply the following questions to examine each soft power asset in health diplomacy in Chapter 4:

1. How is the initiative different from a coercion action associated with political inferences, market maneuver, or image fabrication? (risk)
2. Is the initiative deemed attractive, desirable, and legitimate in the recipient country, given the recipient country's social, legal, and political system? (risk)
3. What can help the initiative be sustainable in the long term? (limitation)
4. What is the best strategy to adapt the initiative to the local language and culture? (limitation)

The ROK's Soft Power Assets Pre–COVID-19

In the year before the COVID-19 pandemic, the ROK reached its best overall soft power ranking (SP30, 2019).[2] According to the SP30 index, between 2016 to 2019, the ROK improved its government subindex related to effectiveness and individual freedoms. Meanwhile, the country's extensive tourism campaign, led by K-pop, improved its global ties at the people-to-people level. The ROK continued to excel in its digital platforms and technology enterprise, which were its most well-known soft power assets. The ROK's soft power measures are relatively weak in foreign policy engagement.

In the next two chapters, we summarize the ROK's COVID-19 response strategies and its system and governance foundations, then assess the responses' potential as soft power assets. Ultimately, we sought to assess how the response has contributed to the country's soft power and to provide policy recommendations on the new initiatives for implementation.

---

[2] The SP30 index has five years of data between 2015 and 2019. The ROK's index was 54.3 (20th) in 2015, 51.4 (22nd) in 2016, 58.4 (21st) in 2017, 62.8 (20th) in 2018, and 63.0 (19th) in 2019 (see SP30, 2015–2019).

Chapter 3. The ROK's COVID-19 Initial Response and Its Foundations

In this chapter, we discuss six features of the ROK's success in containing COVID-19 early in the pandemic and its public health system and governance foundations. We identified these factors primarily through a comprehensive literature review, supplemented by stakeholder interviews.

The ROK's Success in Containing COVID-19

In 2020, as the whole world came to a halt to combat the COVID-19 pandemic, each country faced a unique epidemic pattern because of variations in virus transmission routes, sociodemographic factors, and pandemic response strategies. The ROK, because of its geographic proximity, shares a significant amount of trade, business, and tourism traffic with China. When the virus began to spread in China in December 2019, the ROK was one of the first countries, other than China, to detect COVID-19 cases, in January 2020. By February 2020, the ROK had the second-highest number of cases of any country in the world, following China, showing that the new coronavirus was spreading explosively.

However, despite this initial high burden of disease, the ROK was able to quickly reduce the number of new cases and sustained a low mortality rate in the first year of the pandemic, before the vaccines and treatments were available. Compared with other countries or regions that experienced an outbreak in the first six months of the year, the ROK maintained a low case-fatality rate of 1.2 percent during the first outbreak, compared with 9.3 percent in Italy, 7.8 percent in Iran, 4.3 percent in France, and 9.2 percent in New York City. More significantly, the ROK flattened the curve without a large-scale and strict lockdown, which could have led to economic paralysis or social despair. In 2020, the nation's gross domestic product contracted by only 1 percent, compared with 5.3 percent in Japan, 3.7 percent in the United States, and 11.2 percent in the United Kingdom. The overall unemployment rate increased 1 percent relative to the estimated rate before the pandemic (Dyer, 2021).

Many countries emulated the ROK's initial successful COVID-19 strategy, which public health scholars worldwide observed. Using a systematic approach, we scanned 1,863 academic articles published in 2020 and 2021 and fully reviewed 63 articles (see the appendix).[3] This literature review allowed us to summarize the COVID-19 epidemic pattern and identify six characteristics of the pandemic response. We also studied the context of this response, including the ROK's public health infrastructure (as evaluated in the World Health Organization's

---

[3] The search was completed on May 13, 2021.

[WHO's] Joint External Evaluation [JEE] report) and social-ecological system (SES). As Figure 3.1 illustrates, the ROK's strong public health infrastructure, along with its unique social and governance factors, laid the foundation for and contributed to the six features of the successful initial response to and management of the COVID-19 pandemic and the resulting epidemic patterns. We discovered that these foundations were further strengthened in operations during the ROK's 2015 experiences with Middle East respiratory syndrome (MERS) and, hence, included highlights of the ROK policy and the legal changes after MERS.

In the following sections, we first introduce the six characteristics we identified. We then explain how the successful response benefited from the ROK's public health infrastructure, its society and governing systems, and its experience with MERS. Finally, we compare the ROK's pandemic response with those of other Asian countries to further understand its successful pandemic management.

Figure 3.1. A Multifaceted Framework of Pandemic Response Readiness Helps Explain the ROK's Successful Initial Response to COVID-19 in 2020

Public health infrastructure (JEE)	**Strengthened by 2015 MERS legacies**	**ROK pandemic response**	**Epidemic patterns**
• National coordination and health finance • Testing, surveillance, and contact tracing • Supply chain and workforce • Risk communications	• Revisions on the infectious disease law • Establishment of new Emergency Operation Center and communication team • Investment in infectious disease diagnostic technology • Establishment of emergency use authorization program for test kits • Preparations of citizens to comply	• A sensitive pandemic alert system and pandemic preparation • A centralized hierarchical response system • COVID-19 national testing strategy • Stringent infection tracing and containment strategies • Information communication and technology applications • A two-track COVID-19 hospital triage system	• Low incidence rate • Low infection rate • Low death rate • Low mortality rate • Low community transmission rate • Limited community outbreaks
SES • Social factors • Resources • Governance style • Citizen's trust			

NOTE: The blue box highlights elements learned from the response to MERS.

Six Features of the Initial Response to COVID-19

A Sensitive Pandemic Alert System and Pandemic Preparation

The ROK government initiated its first infectious disease alert (Level 1) on January 3, 2020, four days after the China National Health Commission reported a cluster of cases of pneumonia of unknown origin to WHO (Dyer, 2021).[4] Soon after, identification of the first imported case, at

---

[4] The four-level alert system consists of levels: level 1, the government begins to monitor the epidemic; level 2, a case enters the country, and the government activates cooperation system; level 3, infection spreads to other areas,

Incheon International Airport on January 20, 2020, triggered Level 2 (Why Korea Rushed . . . ,"
2020; Chen et al., 2021; Zhu and Liu, 2021). In the following days, quarantine and screening at
the country's border expanded, while epidemiologic studies were conducted to trace the contacts
of the index case (Moradi and Vaezi, 2020). By January 30, 2020, when WHO first labeled
COVID-19 as a public health emergency, the ROK government had already raised the national
alert to Level 3 and allocated U.S. $17 million for pandemic emergency funds and U.S. $1.6
billion for reserve funds. On February 23, 2020, detection of the first local outbreak triggered a
Level 4 alert (the highest level). In summary, the early alert allowed the ROK government to
enhance early case screening at borders, develop diagnostic tools, establish response plans, and
secure human resources for the epidemic control before its first outbreak (Oh et al., 2020). One
public health expert we interviewed commented that experience with 2015 MERS epidemic
prompted the early initiation of the ROK's unique four-level infectious disease alert system.

A Centralized Hierarchical Response System to Coordinate Pandemic Resource Allocation and Risk Communication

As soon as the Level 4 alert activated the pandemic response protocols, the ROK prime
minister, together with two other ministers, established the Central Disaster and Safety
Countermeasure Headquarters and Control Tower (Lee et al., 2021). This headquarters was
instrumental in mobilizing medical resources, building an emergency public-private partnership
for producing supplies, and communicating with the public.

For example, to prevent a shortage of face masks at the beginning of the pandemic, the
headquarters directly managed the production, logistics, and distribution of masks through a five-
day production rotation system in the factories while also banning exports. Rations of two N-95
or KF-94 masks were issued by headquarters when there were shortages of filtration masks for
health professionals. Throughout the pandemic, the Health Insurance Review and Assessment
Service ran a digitalized pharmacy health data portal, which enabled monitoring of mask prices
and restrictions. By April 2020, 11.1 million masks were being provided daily. Two months
later, ROK local production met more than 80 percent of the mask demands in the country
(Jeong et al., 2020; Arora, Rajput, and Changotra, 2020; Kim and Ashihara, 2020; Choi et al.,
2020).

Communications from headquarters during the pandemic were direct and consistent and
based on real-time data (Jeong et al., 2020). The platforms included daily press conferences, real-
time text-message alerts, and smartphone applications (Zeng, Bernardo, and Havins, 2020; Kang
et al., 2020). One article commented that the ROK government's effective risk communications
strengthened a collective society mindset and supported an unprecedented high level of
compliance among citizens with public health interventions, such as mask-wearing, social

---

and the response system is initiated; and level 4, the nationwide response system is activated. See Moradi and Vaezi,
2020.

distancing, and quarantine (Lee and Lee, 2020). As a result, no national lockdown was initiated, and localized lockdowns were implemented only in highly infected areas (Ling et al., 2021), while panic buying and hoarding of masks were rare. In our interviews, several experts commented that the ROK has a high level of public compliance while remaining a democratic country in which elections and demonstrations were not suppressed, even when stringent public health measures were implemented.

COVID-19 National Testing Strategy

The ROK's effective national COVID-19 testing strategy was instrumental to its pandemic response success (Zeng, Bernardo, and Havins, 2020; Kang et al., 2020). The early and rapid expansion of COVID-19 testing was built on two critical developments in the ROK, which were prompted by its 2015 experience with MERS: (1) the ROK Ministry of Science and Information and Communication Technology's U.S. $25-million investment in infectious disease diagnostic technology in 2017[5], which established a key public and private partnership for diagnostic testing (Shuren and Stenzel, 2021), and (2) the establishment of an agency-led emergency use authorization program to fast-track test kits during pandemics (Shuren and Stenzel, 2021, Lee et al., 2021, Oh et al., 2020). Together with the government's guaranteed purchase to minimize financial risk, more than 20 companies started to develop and produce polymerase chain reaction testing kits at a time when only four cases had been identified in the ROK, in January 2020.

On February 7, 2020, the tests were approved under the emergency use authorization, and the testing kits were distributed nationally, and the number of free screening clinics expanded from 288 to 663 by April 20, 2020 (Arora, Rajput, and Changotra, 2020; Ling et al., 2021).[6] These clinics had also learned a lesson from MERS, when widespread infection at hospitals was a main driver of the outbreak. This time, the ROK government swiftly established three types of safe testing setting: drive-through testing, testing booths at clinics, and walk-through testing centers (Lee and Lee, 2020; Kim and Ashihara, 2020; Arora, Rajput, and Changotra, 2020; Choi et al., 2020; Heo et al., 2020; Chen et al., 2021). To protect individuals' privacy, testing was also offered anonymously, with results provided through phone calls with no name record (Choi et al., 2020).

Stringent Infection Tracing and Containment Strategies

Large-scale testing alone is not sufficient to contain an outbreak unless combined with other public health measures, such as social distancing, self-quarantine, contact tracing, and patient

---

[5] Unless otherwise indicated, all dollar amounts are in U.S. dollars.

[6] An ROK health economist pointed out that the ROK's testing technology and capacity had been high pre–COVID-19, and some even considered this to be overcapacity. The ROK's national health insurance system provides disproportionate reimbursement for the testing in clinical settings, which protects the robust testing infrastructure in the country.

isolation (Jeong et al., 2020). To contain the first outbreak in February, the ROK investigation team tested almost all members of the Shincheonji temple, where transmission began, and mapped and tested their contacts, while requesting that all Daegu citizens voluntarily self-quarantine for at least two weeks (Choi et al., 2020). Contact tracing in large clusters was handled by national, provincial, and city government offices, while county officials handled contact tracing and quarantine in family units (Oh et al., 2020). Later, labor-intensive contact tracing was replaced by less-labor-intensive digital contact tracing.

The ROK also implemented a stringent quarantine and isolation strategy in the first year of the pandemic. International travelers who tested positive at walk-through screening centers at the airport were immediately escorted to a hospital or Living Treatment Center for isolation (Kim et al., 2021). Those with negative test results were asked to self-isolate for 14 days at home or at designated hotels and to be retested. Violation of the Quarantine Act and Infectious Disease Control and Prevention Act resulted in a prison sentence or a heavy fine. All people who were COVID-19 positive were required to check in with health authorities once a day for two weeks. Those who failed to do so within two days of arrival would receive a direct call from health authorities. Electronic wristbands (with consent) were required for anyone who violated self-isolation rules (Choi et al., 2020; Heo et al., 2020).

Information and Communication Technology Applications

Such a stringent tracing and containment strategy would not have been sustainable over time if the ROK government had not deployed ICT applications (Heo et al., 2020). Table 3.1 itemizes the ICT technologies used for various segments of the pandemic response. For instance, all arrivals into ports of entry were required to download a government-mandated Self-Quarantine Safety Protection software application, which allowed authorities to monitor their locations using the Global Positioning System. Private enterprises (e.g., telecommunications and credit card companies) supported the COVID-19 Epidemiological Investigation Support System, which allows contact tracers to identify the transmission routes of an infected individual using Global Positioning System locations, closed-circuit television, and credit card transactions.

Table 3.1. The ROK's Digital Technologies for Containment Strategy

Measures	Alerting and Warning		Epidemiological Investigation		Quarantine of Contacts			Social Distancing	Mask-Wearing
	Pandemic Information for the Public	Infection Risk to Potential Contacts	Contacts Tracing	Detection of Imported	Border Control and Tracking	Voluntary or Involuntary Isolation	Case-Finding		
Cellular Broadcasting Service	✓	✓						✓	✓
Artificial Intelligence Chatbot	✓	✓	✓	✓		✓	✓	✓	
Smart Working								✓	
Remote Education								✓	
Diagnosis Application			✓	✓		✓	✓		
Quarantine Application			✓		✓	✓	✓		
Smart Quarantine Information System				✓	✓		✓	✓	
Epidemiological Investigation Support System			✓	✓			✓	✓	

SOURCE: Heo et al., 2020.

NOTE: Blue boxes indicate which technologies addressed each measure.

In addition to case tracking and management, ICT also supported government emergency communications, remote work, remote education, and telemedicine. Other ICTs were widely used in supporting research on drug repurposing, artificial-intelligence guided medicine development, and online sales of agricultural products (Lee et al., 2021; Arora, Rajput, and Changotra, 2020). Insights from expert interviews emphasized that the public has accepted government use of individuals' personal data during the pandemic, as permitted by the revised infectious disease law that was enacted pre–COVID-19. The current pandemic strategy validated the use of ICT to facilitate infectious disease control and help more people accept disease surveillance during the pandemic.

A Two-Track COVID-19 Hospital Triage System

The ROK also successfully maintained a functioning health care system during the pandemic. The ROK had a strong health system with a high density of hospital beds and resources (10.6 beds per 100,000 residents) and an established single-payer universal health care system pre–COVID-19 (Ling, 2021). Nonetheless, the first outbreak of COVID-19 caused a shortage of health care workers in Daegu (Choi He-suk, 2020). Health care workers from the army, public health, and other areas had to be dispatched to Daegu to help (Sejin Choi, 2020).

The ROK subsequently redesigned health service provision at the national level to operate the COVID-19 health system and the non–COVID-19 health system. A national-level coordination center managed the flow of COVID-19 patients to hospitals or, if needed, to other provinces, while patients with non–COVID-19 conditions were sent to "system safety guaranteed hospitals" (Oh et al., 2020). COVID-19 patients were further categorized based on risk level:

1. Critically ill patients were sent to established university hospitals equipped with negative-pressure intensive-care units and staffed with respiratory and infectious disease specialists.
2. Patients with severe COVID-19 but not critically ill were transferred to a general hospital with negative-pressure units and specialists.
3. Patients with mild to moderate cases were sent to use nonhospital beds in training centers and dormitories, which were converted into temporary clinics as accommodation support centers (also called community treatment centers, residential treatment centers, or living treatment centers) (Yang, Kim, and Hwang, 2020; Kang et al., 2020).

Foundations of Success

The literature and expert opinions have often credited lessons learned from the response to MERS—and the subsequent amendments to the ROK's infectious disease law—for the success of the response to COVID-19, as illustrated in the highlighted section of Figure 3.1. In particular, the infectious disease law enabled the use of ICT and closed-circuit television for epidemiological investigation during pandemics. The revised law also helped sustain the funding for an infectious disease surveillance system and public health workforce training. After MERS, the ROK also established a new emergency operation center, pathogen detection and analysis division, and communication team in the Korea Disease Control and Prevention Agency (KCDC); increased the number of intensive-care unit beds; and clarified public-private collaboration protocols during a pandemic (Kang et al., 2020; Dongarwar and Salihu, 2021; Oh et al., 2020; Choi et al., 2020; Lee et al., 2021). The three T strategy (testing, tracing, and treatment) and the four T strategy (three T plus transparency) were considered key components of the ROK's COVID-19 response.[7] These comprehensive improvements following the MERS epidemic established the public health foundation for the response to COVID-19 in 2020.

ROK's Public Health Infrastructure as Foundations for COVID-19 Response

As a result of these improvements, the ROK ranked high in its pandemic preparedness in multiple global infectious disease control indexes prior to the first outbreak of COVID-19 (Moore, Gelfeld, and Okunogbe, 2017).[8] As Figure 3.1 illustrates, the well-established public health infrastructure was the fundamental component that enabled the ROK to implement effective initial response and pandemic management strategies. In 2017, ROK implemented WHO's JEE. JEE provides the most-comprehensive evaluation of a country's health security infrastructure and is based on a standard process involving both in-country expert opinions and an international expert panel (WHO, 2018). The report contains 48 indicators to examine 19 factors in the four domains of health security (prevent, detect, respond, and other).

For this project, we selected indicators in the four domains of capacity that are most relevant to the COVID-19 response (see Table 3.1), including national coordination and health finance; testing, surveillance, and contact tracing; supplies and workforce management; and risk communication. Under each domain, we compared the ROK's average score of the subdomain's levels of capacity with that of Indonesia—the other Asian country that completed JEE—and to that of the United States.

Table 3.2 shows that the ROK's pandemic response system pre–COVID-19 received higher scores than those of Indonesia and United States in many items. The table also highlights the ROK's superb readiness in its emergency operation programs and activation mechanisms; its laboratory capability in specimen transportation, testing, reporting, and supporting the surveillance networks; and its public health workforce training and dispatch. Even the relatively weak items, with a score of 3 in the report, such as partner communication and communication engagement with communities and resource mapping, were strengthened during the COVID-19 response under the strong leadership of the command tower.

---

[7] Stakeholder interview with an ROK public health expert.

[8] The ROK ranked ninth in the Johns Hopkins Global Health Security Index ("Global Health Security Index," undated) and 16th in the RAND Pandemic Vulnerability Score.

Table 3.2. Joint External Evaluation Indicators That Are Most Relevant to the COVID-19 Response

Attributes	ROK	Indonesia	USA
National pandemic preparedness coordination and plans[a]			
National public health emergency preparedness and response plan is developed and implemented	5	3	5
Priority public health risks and resources are mapped and utilized	3	2	4
Capacity to activate emergency operations	5	3	5
Emergency operation center operating procedures and plans	4	2	4
Emergency operations program	5	3	4
Routine capacities established at points of entry	5	4	4
Effective public health response at points of entry	5	4	5
Testing, surveillance, and contact tracing[b]			
Laboratory testing for detection of priority diseases	5	4	5
Specimen referral and transport system	5	4	4
Effective modern point-of-care and laboratory-based diagnostics	5	3	5
Laboratory quality system	4	3	5
Indicator- and event-based surveillance systems	5	3	5
Interoperable, interconnected, electronic real-time report system	5	3	3
Integration and analysis of surveillance data	5	2	5
Syndromic surveillance systems	4	4	4
System for efficient reporting to the Food and Agriculture Organization of the United Nations, World Organisation for Animal Health, and WHO	5	3	5
Reporting network and protocols in country	5	3	4
Health finance, supply chain, and workforce[c]			
Legislation, laws, regulations, administrative requirements, policies in place are sufficient for implementation of IHR	5	3	5
The State can demonstrate that it has adjusted and aligned its domestic legislation/policies to enable compliance with IHR	5	3	5
Human resources available to implement IHR core capacity	5	3	5
Applied epidemiology training program in place	5	4	5
Workforce strategy	4	3	4
Risk communications[d]			
Risk communication systems (plans, mechanisms, etc.)	4	3	4
Internal and partner communication and coordination	3	3	5
Public communication	4	4	4

Attributes	ROK	Indonesia	USA
Communication engagement with affected communities	3	4	3
Dynamic listening and rumor management	4	4	4

SOURCES: WHO, 2016; WHO, 2017a; WHO, 2017b; attribute wordings adapted from these sources.

NOTES: The scores are

1 = No capacity: Attributes of a capacity are not in place.

2 = Limited capacity: Attributes of a capacity are in development stage.

3 = Developed capacity: Attributes of a capacity are in place; however, sustainability has not been ensured.

4 = Demonstrated capacity: Attributes are in place, sustainable for a few more years.

5 = Sustainable capacity: Attributes are functional and sustainable, and the country is supporting other countries in its implementation.

[a] Includes items R1.1-1.2, R2.1-2.3, PoE.1-2 in the JEE report.

[b] Includes items D1.1-1.4, D2.1-2.4, D3.2-3.2 in the JEE report.

[c] Includes items P1.1-1.2, D4.1-4.3 in the JEE report.

[d] Includes items R5.1-5.5 in the JEE report.

16

The ROK epidemic experts we interviewed during COVID-19 confirmed the JEE report findings. In addition, several highlighted the importance of local public health centers and national health insurance coverage as foundations for the pandemic response. Even though the local governments initially followed the KCDC guidelines strictly, they were able to be more innovative later in the pandemic as they gained more knowledge and confidence on COVID-19. Such capacity at the community level was strengthened by a long-term development in the community health care workforce, vast amounts of government and private funding in public and private hospitals, amended laws on disease control, establishment of a risk communication division in government, and high cell phone usage for e-messaging from government.

ROK's Society and Governing Systems as Foundations for COVID-19 Response

In addition to the public health system, a country's social, physical, economic, and governance factors also affect its pandemic response (Suhud et al., 2020; Ling et al., 2021). We therefore looked into the SES framework and its application on analyzing COVID-19 initial responses (McGinnis and Ostrom, 2014). Suhud et al. and Ling et al. (2020, 2021) explored the multifaceted social, physical, and governance factors that affected Asian countries' success level in combating COVID-19 (Suhud et al., 2020; Ling et al., 2021). Table 3.3 summarizes rankings on key factors, including population density, social homogeneity, civil trust, economic development, and governing style, both for the ROK and, as a comparison, Indonesia.

As Figure 3.1 and Table 3.3 illustrate, the ROK possesses several important social, resource, and governance attributes that helped the country manage the COVID-19 pandemic well despite its disadvantage in terms of high population density. Although having high levels of SES factors is not a complete solution for the pandemic, such attributes as social homogeneity, superb health care and technology resources; experience with MERS; significant economic power; and a governing style that includes strict penalties for policy violations were contributing factors.

Other reports support the ROK's success in establishing transparent and effective government-public communications post-MERS, which helped in the COVID-19 response (Chen et al., 2021; Zeng, Bernardo, and Havins, 2020; Jeong et al., 2020; Ling et al., 2021; Kim and Ashihara, 2020; Choi et al., 2020). Stakeholders we interviewed also pointed out that close collaboration between public and private entities during the MERS pandemic had laid the foundation for effective public-private collaboration during the COVID-19 pandemic. The ROK's recent MERS experience also prepared citizens to comply with government guidelines and measures, such as quarantine policies, and to accept the collection and public use of private data.

Table 3.3. Social-Ecological System Factors Relevant to COVID-19 Response

Attributes	Definition	Hypothetical Relation to COVID-19	ROK	Indonesia
Population density	Number of populations per land area	Higher density can increase transmission rate	High	Low
Social homogeneity	Race/ethnicity, language diversity	Higher homogeneity may increase cooperation level and collective interests	High	Medium
Trust	Trust between citizens and government	Trust in government capacity and communication increases compliance with government rules	Medium	Medium
Health facilities[a]	Density of physician and hospital beds	An overwhelmed health care system can cause excessive deaths	High	Low
Technology and manufacturing	Technology infrastructure	These provide necessary material for timely and sufficient detection, isolation, and treatment options	High	High
Economic power	Gross national income per capita of a country	Economic power aids financial relief and facility support	High	Medium
Top-down leadership	Governing style	Top-down leadership seems to boost compliant behaviors	Medium	Medium
Strict penalty	Punishment or fine	Penalties discourage self-interest	High	Medium

SOURCE: Ling et al., 2021.
[a] According to Table 8 in Ling et al., 2021, density of physicians (per 10,000) was 3.777 for Indonesia in 2018 and 23.661 for South Korea in 2018, and the density of hospital beds (per 10,000) was 10.4 for Indonesia in 2017 and 124.3 for South Korea in 2018.

Experts we interviewed added that the high level of compliance among the general public in the ROK is similar to that in other East Asian countries, such as Japan, China, and Vietnam, which are societies that value a collective responsibility and public goods more than individual freedom and interests. These factors all contributed to the high level of individual adherence to the public prevention protocols KCDC recommended (Arora, Rajput, and Changotra, 2020; Lee and Lee, 2020; Lee et al., 2021; Oh et al., 2020a).

Reflection on the Gaps in Pandemic Responses in Some Other Asian Countries

As a comparison, we also looked into India and Indonesia's approaches to COVID-19 to reflect on the challenges and barriers for disease containment. Our comprehensive literature review did not provide many in-depth studies on this topic at the time of our research. During stakeholder interviews, experts from other Asian countries noted additional gaps in their countries' pandemic responses that further highlight the ROK's successful initial response to COVID-19. For example, experts mentioned that India had the technology for contact tracing and that Indonesia was able to develop the technology, but both countries encountered implementation challenges related to their decentralized governing systems, stigma around COVID-19, and lack of consensus on privacy concerns during a pandemic. In addition, limited public data-sharing practices in India and Indonesia hindered private companies' and the public's access to the real-time pandemic situation and slowed the distribution of much-needed medical resources and personal protective equipment (PPE).

The private health care system in India was fragmented and lacked guidance. Indonesia used help from the military, police, and private sectors but was still incapable of fulfilling the needs of testing. Also, both countries lacked isolation facilities and quality-assured national and regional laboratories, and the workforces were not sufficiently trained to combat the COVID-19 pandemic.

Although India had a national law and legal act that allowed the federal government to lead and implement quarantine and surveillance, the authorities managing public health were largely decentralized and lacked effective coordination. Indonesia, on the other hand, lacked effective surveillance and a sensitive disease alert system and had a weak health care system prior to COVID-19.

India strove for private-sector multilateral cooperation but has not yet achieved it because of the lack of global and regional platforms for collaboration during the early years of COVID-19. Indonesia suffers from a different issue. Some experts suggested that, while the country is a big market and has a lot of potential for international collaboration on global health, the Indonesian public is historically skeptical of partnerships with other countries in the region and with big companies in the private sector.

In contrast, ROK's strong capacity for testing, well-established health system, highly effective public-private collaboration, high citizen compliance, and relevant laws dating from the response to MERS allowed the country to handle the crisis successfully.

Chapter 4. Soft Power Assets and Risks from the ROK's COVID-19 Response

The ROK's COVID-19 response success demonstrated multiple attractive features, such as effective government-enterprise collaboration, outstanding digital infrastructure and applications, competent government communication and centralized command, a relatively well-trained government and public health workforce, a collective yet democratic culture, and resilience in health care capacity during a crisis. Many of these features could be leveraged to build soft power through health diplomacy. In this chapter, we explore the potential soft power assets derived from this success that might be used for health diplomacy.

The ROK's Soft Power Assets and Activities

We first map potential soft power assets and activities and the associated risks onto SP30's six domains of soft power assets (Table 4.1). We will then complement this analysis with interview feedback from Indian and Indonesian experts on their countries' gap in COVID-19 responses and the ROK experts' views on building soft power.

Digital Soft Power

Digital soft power refers to a country's digital infrastructure and capabilities in digital diplomacy. This was the ROK's highest-ranked soft power subdomain asset pre–COVID-19. The ROK is well respected for having built a robust infrastructure to enhance e-government and e-participation. The ROK's COVID-19 strategy success multiplied the value of this asset by setting a good example of how digital technology can be used in a pandemic containment strategy for alerting and warning; epidemiological investigation; quarantine and isolation management; and enhancing case-finding, social distancing, and mask-wearing policies (see Chapter 3). A German report found that technological capabilities have been the most important factor boosting the ROK's image, especially as the country demonstrated its ability to conduct large-scale testing (Amiri, 2022).

The main risk associated with this soft power asset involves concerns about privacy issues, authoritarianism, and other legal and political issues related to the system of governance. These negatively affected public opinion in some, though not all, countries (Greitens, 2020). The ROK's role as a democratic country that has a pandemic infectious disease law allowing the government to use private data for digital tracing provides a counter to the concern about authoritarianism (Lim and Sziarto, 2020).

Table 4.1. ROK Soft Power Assets and Risks from COVID-19 Responses

Domain	Potential Assets	Potential Activities	Potential Risks of Applying Assets[a]
Digital resources	The ROK's application of digital technologies in disease surveillance, contact tracing, information dissemination, and quarantine and isolation monitoring demonstrated its robust digital infrastructure (WiFi and cell-phone coverage and usage) and innovative applications. Countries have been impressed with the ROK's technology advancement and are interested in learning about its application in health.	• Providing technical support on ICT applications in health and governance • Providing technical training • Collaborating on research • Transferring technology and donating digital devices • Contributing to regional supply and infrastructure	• Concerns exist about government violation of citizens' privacy. • This can be perceived a market coercion or competition. • Digital infrastructure–building leads to environmental concerns, financial concerns (funding gap and increasing debt), and sustainability risks.
Private-enterprise resources	ROK enterprises are innovative and powerful. The ROK's pandemic response law requires private industry's cooperation. A strong public-private partnership led to the development and production of an early testing kit. The ROK joined the market leadership group of Access to COVID-19 Tools (ACT) Accelerator (ACT-A) to support ACT diagnostic kit production. ROK private companies also joined forces with the government to implement COVID-19 control–related applications.	• Building a global or regional biomedical product supply chain and manufacturing hub for vaccines, diagnostic kits, PPE, and treatments • Providing technical consultation on legal frameworks for public-private partnership in public health • Collaborating on research and development collaborations	• Are the ROK's enterprise operation culture and norms desirable for other countries? • Collaborations with ROK enterprise may be considered coercion. • Language and cultural barriers can hamper collaboration.
Education and labor-market resources	ROK universities are not well known in the world. Highlighting their role in the COVID-19 response will spur new collaborations and help promote building of a regional knowledge and training center. ROK university medical centers were instrumental in providing COVID-19 care; universities hosted career training for local government public health professionals.	• Joining regional infectious disease prevention and response knowledge and expert networks • Providing in-country demonstration and training • Providing ROK-based training for professionals and foreign students • Developing exchange scholar programs and joint scientific research	• Concerns exist about whether funding will be sustainable. • Language and culture can be barriers unless languages other than Korean can be used in parts of the universities. • Fears exist about brain drain—that professionals from developing countries will leave their home countries.

21

Domain	Potential Assets	Potential Activities	Potential Risks of Applying Assets[a]
Culture resources	COVID-19 highlighted the ROK's high level of civil trust, culture of mask wearing, and collective society culture (focused on caring for the community, not just self), while also remaining an active democratic country.	• Engaging in civil-society visiting programs • Engaging in foreign student exchange programs • Using music, storytelling, and entertainment channels to highlight ROK culture	• The ROK's highly collective culture could be viewed as working against personal freedom and would not be desirable in some countries. • Explanations should target the rationale for the collective actions during COVID-19.
Engagement activities	COVID-19 prompted the ROK to be more engaged in global health assistance programs. Activities include medical PPE donations; a U.S. $200-million commitment to COVID vaccine funding in 2021 and 2022 at the Group of Seven; donations of U.S. $25 million to Global Fund to Fight AIDS, Tuberculosis and Malaria and U.S. $9 million to the Coalition for Epidemic Preparedness Innovations; and midterm planning to include collaboration to fight COVID-19.	• Increasing official development assistance (ODA) associated with health • Increasing support to and collaboration with multilateral health organizations • Donating vaccines and PPE • Increasing humanitarian aid	• Concerns exist about whether such government engagement efforts will be sustainable post–COVID-19 and whether all ministries would consider global health assistance a priority post COVID-19. • Questions exist about whether any of the assistance programs would be interpreted as being coercive. • Would language and culture be a barrier?
Government	The ROK COVID-19 response command center model and the national pandemic alert system fully demonstrated the government's effectiveness. The ROK also modeled the rule of law: Infectious disease law updates after MERS were instrumental in the COVID-19 response. The ROK also demonstrated that a collective culture can coexist with democracy: Elections and protests were protected during the pandemic.	• Government program demonstration in mass media • Invite other countries' delegation teams for visits • Invite short-term exchange staff	• The ROK government and its governing style are not as well known in the outside world as its technology and private enterprises. • Would the efficiency and top-down style be desirable in other countries? • Will the failure to reduce gender inequality and boost fast-declining fertility affect the ROK's soft power? • Concerns exist about whether the ROK is seeking to influence other countries' domestic policy.

22

SOURCES: McClory, 2015; McClory, 2019.
[a] Based on the four risk categories from Chapter 2: coercion, desirability, sustainability, and adaptability.

As with other infrastructure projects, digital infrastructure–building is much needed in developing countries. Yet, such a project is often geared toward long-term benefits rather than short-term profit, and the recipient countries and the ROK need to reach agreement on environmental protection, finance plans, and security concerns. The ROK can also provide technical support to multilateral international development agencies, such as the World Bank Group.

Enterprise Soft Power

Enterprise soft power refers to the attractiveness of a country's economic model, business friendliness, and capacity for innovation. One highlight of the ROK's initial success in responding to COVID-19 is the ample supply of testing kits before the first outbreak in February 2020. The speed of testing kit development, approval, and production relied on ROK biotechnology companies' innovation, dedication, and capacity. Such a good reputation can promote the ROK's and other countries' business-to-business connections and collaborations. The ROK contributed an additional U.S. $1 million to Unitaid in 2020 to increase access to COVID-19 diagnostics through ACT-A. ROK joined ACT-A as a Facilitation Council member, providing strategic advice and guidance to ACT-A, and is one of nine countries—with the United States, China, India, Russia, Brazil, Indonesia, South Africa, and Mexico—in the "market leader group" (Donor Tracker, undated).

The risk inherent of this soft power asset is concern about whether collaboration with the ROK enterprise might be perceived as a form of economic coercion. The ROK already supplies a large market in electronics and automobiles in many developing countries (e.g., Samsung). Adding the biomedical industry to the list can follow a similar practice and ensure that the recipient country can benefit from newly created jobs and technology transfers.

Education Soft Power

Education soft power represents the level of human capital in a country, its contribution to scholarship, and its attractiveness to international students. Although the ROK's universities are destinations for many international students in South Asia, its public health and medical specialties are not well known around the world. During the pandemic, most of the COVID-19 patients who needed negative pressure rooms and intensive care were cared for by teaching hospitals in the ROK. The experience gained from COVID-19's successful strategy can serve as a new platform to attract students and scholars.

The risk of this soft power asset concerns the sustainability of the large amount of funding needed to develop universities and training centers as hubs of knowledge post–COVID-19. On the other hand, tuition revenue can be a long-term gain if the initiatives can boost the reputations of ROK educational institutions. Barriers from the unique language and culture can be overcome if other languages (e.g., English) can be used for international programs and if more cultural exchange programs are installed in the education system.

Culture Soft Power

Culture soft power refers to the global reach and appeal of a nation's cultural outputs, both in pop culture and high culture. Cultural attributes, such as social acceptance of mask-wearing and caring for the community (not just self), played a positive role in the ROK's COVID-19 response. Such cultural attributes can elicit good will and collaboration in countries with a similar cultural background (mostly in East Asia). However, highlighting such cultural attributes in countries that focus on individual freedom may risk backlash.

In stakeholder interviews, experts pointed out that the ROK's success in technology development and industrialization is well known to the average Indian, as is the ROK's strength in gadgets, telemedicine, and pharmaceuticals. Indians are also very familiar with ROK pop culture. However, most Asian countries have very limited knowledge of the ROK's success in managing COVID-19. Only one expert mentioned having had one seminar on COVID-19 management in Indonesia's embassy in the ROK.

Engagement

Engagement refers to the strength of a country's diplomatic network and its contribution to global engagement and development. The ROK is the 16th largest donor country in the Organisation for Economic Co-operation and Development, spending 0.14 percent of its gross national income on overseas development funding (Donor Tracker, undated). ROK experts identified this area as one in which the ROK lags behind peer East Asian countries, such as Japan and China. However, the COVID-19 crisis has helped the ROK government set global health as a priority issue in its Midterm Strategy for Development Cooperation (2021–2025) (Donor Tracker, undated). The following multipronged approach was set: (1) ODA to health to increase by 21 percent from U.S. $238 million in 2020 to U.S. $288 million in 2021; (2) minimizing the impact of COVID-19 in partner countries; (3) strengthening and developing the health and medical systems of partner countries; (4) building the infectious disease response capacity in partner countries; and (5) enhancing the ROK's leadership of and contributions to multilateral international organizations, such as the United Nations (UN), WHO, and the UN Educational, Scientific and Cultural Organization. The ROK also seeks to further expand the linkages between its foreign policies, such as the New Northern Policy and the New Southern Policy,[9] and its policies on development cooperation.

The ROK's engagement trajectory on soft power has raised two concerns. One is about the sustainability of a long-term commitment on global health, given the country's lack of tradition and experience in outreach and alliance-building (according to expert interviews); the other

---

[9] The New Northern Policy has focused on strengthening ties with Russia, Mongolia, the countries of Central Asia, and Eastern Europe, while the New Southern Policy is directed at Southeast Asia and India (Botto, 2021).

involves conflicting priorities among different government ministries and the required buy-in from the citizens.

Regarding the first concern, a key question is whether the ROK government's commitment to global vaccine equity will last beyond 2022 post–COVID-19. Another question is whether the ROK government will continue to invest in biomedical research, the pharmaceutical and medical device industries, and international collaborations over the long term. Regarding the second concern, while soft power may be on the main agenda of the Ministry of Foreign Affairs, other ministries (Ministry of Health and Ministry of Finance, for example) may be keen to solve domestic issues on containing the spread of COVID-19 and revitalizing the economy rather than prioritizing global influence. The discord among the ministries can create barriers for the operationalization of the COVID-19–related engagement when multiple ministries would need to collaborate on training, facility building, and budget planning. The new president and his cabinet may have to show clear signals on the trajectory of the overseas development policy.

Governing Style and Effectiveness

Government style refers to the country leadership's commitment to freedom, human rights, and democracy and to the quality of political institutions. Before COVID-19, the ROK government was not considered particularly attractive on government-style issues compared with its prominent reputation on technology and enterprise. The COVID-19 response in the ROK helped bring global attention to the ROK government's effectiveness in containing the outbreak early on and maintaining low incidence in the first year. The government's ability to respond to COVID-19 by setting up an early national pandemic alert, using a centralized command center model to coordinate resources and patient care, and building a public-private partnership for testing were emulated by other countries. During the COVID-19 pandemic, the ROK's infectious disease law, which was updated after the MERS epidemic in 2015, became well known and built the foundation for the government's use of citizens' private data for disease tracing. A recent UN, WHO, and ROK joint evaluation of the country's pandemic preparedness found that the country's disaster response system is highly competent (WHO, 2017a).

The barriers to promoting the ROK's government style as soft power may come from the fact that a country's governing style is often deeply rooted in its unique history and culture and, therefore, hard to change. The ROK government style is democratic but also top-down and centralized. For example, the central ROK government appoints deputy executives at the local government level. These executives often follow instructions from the central government closely and have limited authority to make policy. This government structure is helpful for top-down command in disaster settings, but its success may not easily translate to larger federal-style governing systems.

Chapter 5. Policy Recommendations and Conclusion

Policy Recommendations

As the case studies illustrate, many governments were failing to create effective pandemic solutions because of a lack of well-established health systems, testing capacity, and centralized coordination in the face of the COVID-19 pandemic's destructive path in 2020. The ROK's COVID-19 response model, which is based on the confluence of communal culture, a strong public health foundation, and democratic institutions, offers a powerful example of success in responding to a pandemic and can benefit the nation's brand-building post–COVID-19. As a result, the ROK has an opportunity to promote its image and status in the global health and foreign policy hierarchy. In an increasingly interconnected world, where health is directly linked to economy and security, the ROK's new administration should carefully assess the benefits and risks associated with its COVID-19 response success in terms of health diplomacy.

Recently, the ROK's National Assembly adopted a final ODA budget of KRW 4.4 trillion (U.S. $3.7 billion) for 2022, up 19 percent from that in 2021 and exceeding KRW 4.0 trillion for the first time in history (Donor Tracker, undated). The rise in ODA signaled a commitment to respond to the COVID-19 pandemic using a multilateral strategy. It included a historic U.S. $200 million to the Gavi COVID-19 Vaccine Global Access advance market commitment at the Group of Seven summit in June 2021 to expand the COVID-19 vaccine supply to the low- and middle-income countries. The ROK president, Yoon Seok-yul, campaigned on strengthening the response system to infectious diseases with the aim of making the ROK a vaccine powerhouse. The new Global Health Security Coordination office will—with support from the U.S. Centers for Disease Control and Prevention, the Association of Southeast Asian Nations, and the European Centers for Disease Control—strengthen the ROK's role as a WHO-designated biomanufacturing workforce training hub.

In this context, we offer the following recommendations to support the ROK in building and strengthening its soft power globally beyond the ODA strategy:

- **Build ROK soft power on the nation's advanced biomedical and digital technology. Highlight the COVID-19 success as being rooted in the ROK's powerful technology and enterprises.**

  - This approach highlights the country's technological and industrial strength in biomedical testing and the effective terms of the early development and production of COVID testing. The success is rooted in an effective public-private partnership and the high technical competence of the government and public health workforce. The government can create public health training programs and can partner with businesses to encourage private enterprises to reach out to their global peers for collaboration on innovation and social and public health programs.

- The COVID-19 pandemic underscored the need for innovation in testing and vaccine development. The ROK's success in producing and delivering test kits in a timely manner can be expanded to the production of vaccines and other medical devices. Vaccine and medical supply manufacturers can collaborate with regional partners to expand vaccine capacity and establish the ROK as a global vaccine production hub. The government can assist multilateral organizations in engaging with private companies in the ROK and provide subsidies and incentives for private companies to explore international markets.

- ROK innovation in digital technology and easy access to technologies through the digital infrastructure supported effective risk communication during the COVID-19 pandemic. Other governments may be interested in receiving technical assistance from the ROK to develop digital disease surveillance and communication platforms for public health.

- To avoid the risks that arise with concerns about personal privacy, it is essential to emphasize that the digital technology used in disease tracking and quarantine monitoring relies on citizens' agreement on privacy rights unique to a pandemic era and anchored in the infectious disease law. To minimize the perception of market coercion, manufacturing hubs and alliances should be open to assisting other countries' local economies and supporting technology transfer.

- **Build ROK's soft power through long-term sponsorship of public health science diplomacy.**

  - Building on the success of the COVID-19 response, ROK public health agencies and universities that conduct the training can be modeled as regional pandemic response training centers.

  - ROK public health agencies can also provide steady funding for ROK universities to recruit and train researchers from developing countries to build research and teaching networks. Here the peer-to-peer scientific interactions can enhance the ROK's scientific prowess and reputation.

  - Public health degree programs can be attractive to international students who are interested in learning about the ROK's public health foundation. Long-term government-sponsored scholarships targeting students from specific areas and countries can boost enrollment in these programs.

  - It will be necessary to establish education capacity in many languages, promote cultural openness, and build a long-term financial plan to effectively build soft power through this method. This will require support and collaboration from multiple agencies.

- **Build ROK's soft power through decentralized civil society and governmental exchange programs. ROK's embassies can support linguistic and cultural adaptations.**

  - The ROK's success in the COVID-19 response reflects its unique combination of cultural trends. The ROK's solid, collective compliance was achieved while actively maintaining a democratic political system and institutions. This shows that democracy and citizen trust can coexist in such conditions. This will help the ROK build relationships with countries that favor collective public goods, those that value democratic operations representing the will of the people, and those that favor the rule of law.

- – While government-sponsored civil organization exchange programs can benefit from the involvement of ROK embassy support, a decentralized civil society engagement strategy can reduce concerns about government coercion. Both can aid in the promotion of networks, dialogues, and public diplomacy.

- **Build ROK's soft power through engagement with international multilateral agencies and humanitarian aid.**

  - – COVID-19 has strengthened the ROK's capabilities for health diplomacy, including engagement with global health multilateral organizations (e.g., WHO/ACT, Gavi), and further built alliances with Asia-Pacific countries (via the Association of Southeast Asian Nations). Such global engagement, with the increase in ODA, is poised to increase the ROK's global influence. To maintain this momentum, the ROK will need to sustain the funding and align the interests and priorities of different government ministries.
  - – The ROK should design health care professional training programs that emphasize language and culture diversity to prepare the ROK's physicians and health diplomacy workforce to work in international settings.

Conclusion

As we were finishing this report, we entered the third year of the COVID-19 pandemic. We are acutely aware of the pandemic's long-lasting impact on the health, economy, and security of human society. Policymakers are contemplating when the next pandemic or another natural disaster will strike and whether our society is better prepared. The global health governance agenda places a high priority on the roles of soft power, public diplomacy, and public health preparedness in facilitating a stronger human defenses against new diseases. We believe that both a public health lesson and effective soft power instruments can be drawn from the ROK's initial success in combating the COVID-19 outbreak. This report is anticipated to encourage international collaborations, support the ROK's efforts in forging a strong alliance overseas, and increase health security in Asia and around the globe.

Appendix. Methodology

This report integrated an analysis of findings from a scoping literature review guided by multiple waves of consultations with subject-matter experts in three countries: ROK, India, and Indonesia.

To identify articles, we combined different topic searches from PubMed, including multiple keywords on general pandemic preparedness and specific COVID-19 response and management strategies. Our search strategy on general pandemic preparedness consists of the Medical Subject Heading (MeSH) term "Pandemics" and 17 preparedness-related keywords (limit to title or abstract), such as "planning," "legislation," and "action plan." Similarly, our search strategy on COVID-19 response and management strategies consists of MeSH term "COVID-19" and 42 pandemic-management related keywords (limit to title or abstract), including "laboratory testing," "surveillance system," "contact tracing," "public communication," and "quarantine."

The PubMed search for material related to COVID-19 responses after the year 2020 returned 1,744 academic articles in total. Using Distiller SR, we first reviewed the titles of all identified articles to determine which were off-topic or not related to research. This screening led us to exclude 1,271 documents.

We also conducted a literature search on the Web of Science, specifically focusing on soft power topics and looking only at articles published after 2000 that were cited 15 or more times. Using such keywords as "soft power" and "attractions power," the Web of Science searches returned 119 articles. We have removed 77 off-topic articles through title screening.

We grouped the 515 articles filtered from the title screening into different country groups to prepare for the next stage of screening: ROK, 100; India, 139; Indonesia, 22; China, 145; multiple countries, 38; and other, 71. We then reviewed the abstract for each of the remaining 515 articles and excluded articles that we deemed not to be relevant for purposes. After sorting the articles into high-, medium-, and low-relevance groups, we picked 21 high-priority articles on COVID-19 responses for full-text review. Using Dedoose, we coded each article on the following dimensions: detect (digital technology use, testing and lab capacity, etc.), response (risk communication, private-public partnership, etc.), public health infrastructure (legislation, central response system, etc.), epidemiology, vaccine access and delivery, and country characteristics. We reviewed the full text of all 42 articles related to soft power that emerged from the title screening stage.

In sum, we title-screened 1,863 academic articles on Distiller SR and excluded a total of 1,348 articles from title screening and 452 articles from abstract screening. Figure A.1 outlines the whole screening process.

In addition to searching PubMed, we have also conducted a grey literature search using Google to capture all the news and report articles that are relevant to our research. We ended up including 59 additional references in this report. Although the references do not include any of the 42 soft power articles from our original search, these articles helped us develop grey literature searches, which returned more relevant articles and reports for this research. The analysis of soft power assets used the six SP30 index domains as a conceptual frame.

Figure A.1. Literature Review Selection Process

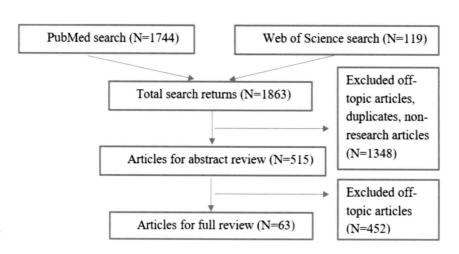

Because we relied on the literature review to supply primary data, we consulted subject-matter experts from the ROK, India, and Indonesia in multiple waves. The first consultation with each expert aimed for confirmations of the keywords and main themes. The second sought feedback after we shared a preliminary draft of findings and the policy recommendations. Experts from India and Indonesia also provided information to supplement the limited literature we could collect. This method ensured that the literature review was conducted under the guidance of the experts in the field and that the policy recommendations are clear and relevant to the target audiences. The experts we consulted included public health experts who could help with our interpretations of the literature on the COVID-19 response and on activities relevant to health diplomacy. These experts were not our primary data points but, rather, were advisors who helped guide the literature review process and provided feedback on what we may have missed or mistaken from the literature.

The following paragraphs describe the rationale for the countries and positions they were chosen from.

The four ROK experts were chosen from academia and have health or public health backgrounds, participated in the pandemic response, and have long collaborated with the government. They helped us understand the extraordinary approaches and the behind-the-scenes discussions during the pandemic. Their input not only shaped our focus as we summarized the unique features of the response but also pointed to the necessary foundations for such a response.

India and Indonesia were chosen as two countries whose initial responses were not as successful as the ROK's. At the time of our literature review, we also found very few comprehensive reports on the COVID-19 responses in India and Indonesia compared to those on the ROK response. Therefore, the experts from these two countries not only gave us feedback on the policy recommendations but also helped us connect the information from the spotty reports and provided supplementary information. In India, our partner helped us identify five experts who were willing to talk to us, including the former minister of the government's response team and representatives of technology companies, community outreach organizations, and public health experts, and who gave us a more complete view of the barriers to the response. From Indonesia, we invited three experts with similar backgrounds.

Before reaching out to experts, we developed outreach materials and interview guides, which were reviewed and approved by the RAND Human Subjects Protection Committee. The initial stakeholder samples were collected through recommendations from our partners, including the Korea Foundation, the Consulate General of the Republic of Korea in Los Angeles, the Asian Century Foundation, and publications.

We conducted the first wave of consultation during September and October 2021. We used open coding to analyze the initial qualitative interview, then axial coding to develop the important features of the ROK's pandemic response. In the second wave, in March 2022, we followed up with experts via emails and collected their feedback on our preliminary analysis and their opinions on our policy suggestions. We then used selective coding to analyze the qualitative data from follow-up interviews to develop our policy recommendations.

Abbreviations

ACT	Access to COVID-19 Tools
ACT-A	Access to COVID-19 Tools Accelerator
COVAX	COVID-19 Vaccines Global Access
COVID-19	coronavirus disease 2019
ICT	information and communication technology
JEE	Joint External Evaluation
KCDC	Korea Disease Control and Prevention Agency
MERS	Middle East respiratory syndrome
ODA	official development assistance
PPE	personal protective equipment
ROK	Republic of Korea
SES	social-ecological system
SP30	Soft Power 30
UN	United Nations
WHO	World Health Organization

References

Amiri, Sohaela, "City Diplomacy: An Introduction to the Forum," *Hague Journal of Diplomacy*, Vol. 17, No. 1, 2022.

Arora, Amarpreet Singh, Himadri Rajput, and Rahil Changotra, "Current Perspective of COVID-19 Spread Across South Korea: Exploratory Data Analysis and Containment of the Pandemic," *Environment, Development and Sustainability*, Vol. 23, No. 5, August 8, 2020.

Botto, Kathryn, *South Korea Beyond Northeast Asia: How Seoul Is Deepening Ties with India and ASEAN*, working paper, Carnegie Endowment for International Peace, 2021.

Bouey, Jennifer, *Implications of US-China Collaborations on Global Health Issues*, RAND Corporation, CT-516, 2019. As of July 25, 2022:
https://www.rand.org/pubs/testimonies/CT516.html

Bouey, Jennifer, *China's Health System Reform and Global Health Strategy in the Context of COVID-19*, RAND Corporation, CT-A321-1, 2020. As of July 25, 2022:
https://www.rand.org/pubs/testimonies/CTA321-1.html

Bourne, Peter G., "A Partnership for International Health Care," *Public Health Reports,* Vol. 93, No. 2, March–April 1978.

Brand Finance, "Global Soft Power Index," webpage, undated. As of July 26, 2022:
https://brandirectory.com/softpower/

Chen, Haiqian, Leiyu Shi, Yuyao Zhang, Xiaohan Wang, and Gang Sun, "Policy Disparities in Response to COVID-19 Between China and South Korea," *Journal of Epidemiology and Global Health*, Vol. 11, No. 2, June 2021.

Choi, Hemin, Wonhyuk Cho, Min-Hyu Kim, and Joon-Young Hur, "Public Health Emergency and Crisis Management: Case Study of SARS-CoV-2 Outbreak," *International Journal of Environmental Research and Public Health*, Vol. 17, No. 11, June 4, 2020.

Choi He-suk, "Nearly 500 Medical Professionals Volunteer for Daegu," *Korea Herald*, February 27, 2020.

Choi, Sejin, "A Hidden Key to COVID-19 Management in Korea: Public Health Doctors," *Journal of Preventive Medicine and Public Health, Vol.* 53, No. 3, April 2020.

Clinton, Hillary Rodham, "Leading Through Civilian Power: Redefining American Diplomacy and Development," *Foreign Affairs*, November–December 2010.

"Coronavirus Pandemic (COVID-19)," webpage, Our World in Data, undated. As of July 26, 2022:
https://ourworldindata.org/coronavirus

Demir, Emre, "China's Wavering COVID-19 Vaccine Diplomacy in Turkey," webpage, Global Voices, August 13, 2021.
https://globalvoices.org/2021/08/13/chinas-wavering-covid-19-vaccine-diplomacy-in-turkey/

Dewi, Sannya Pestari, and Ulul Azmiyati Auliyah, "An Analysis of South Korean TRUST Diplomacy Toward Indonesia in Pandemic Covid-19," *ADI International Conference Series*, Vol. 4, January 2022.

Dongarwar, Deepa, and Hamisu M. Salihu, "Implementation of Universal Health Coverage by South Korea During the COVID-19 Pandemic," *Lancet Regional Health—Western Pacific*, Vol. 7, February 2021.
https://www.ncbi.nlm.nih.gov/pmc/articles/PMC7844349/pdf/main.pdf

Donor Tracker, "South Korea—Global Health," webpage, undated. As of July 26, 2022:
https://donortracker.org/south-korea/globalhealth

Dyer, Paul, "Policy and Institutional Responses to COVID-19: South Korea," Brookings Institution, 2021.
https://www.brookings.edu/research/policy-and-institutional-responses-to-covid-19-south-korea/

Elsayed, Omkolthoum, "Health Diplomacy as a Soft Power: What COVID-19 Has Taught Us," آفاق آسيوية, Vol. 6, No. 6, 2020.

Feinsilver, Julie M., "Cuba's Medical Diplomacy," in Mauricio A. Font, comp., *Changing Cuba/Changing World*, Bildner Center for Western Hemisphere Studies, 2008.

Gauttam, Priya, Bawa Singh, and Jaspal Kaur, "COVID-19 and Chinese Global Health Diplomacy: Geopolitical Opportunity for China's Hegemony?" *Millennial Asia*, Vol. 11, No. 3, 2020.

Global Health Europe, "What Does Global Health Have to Do With Foreign Policy? Hillary Clinton: 'Everything,'" webpage, August 19, 2010.

"Global Health Security Index," homepage, undated. As of July 26, 2022:
https://www.ghsindex.org/

Greitens, Sheena Chestnut, "Surveillance, Security, and Liberal Democracy in the Post-COVID world," *International Organization*, Vol. 74, supplement, December 2020.

Heo, Kyungmoo, Daejoong Lee, Yongseok Seo, and Hyeseung Choi, "Searching for Digital Technologies in Containment and Mitigation Strategies: Experience from South Korea COVID-19," *Annals of Global Health*, Vol. 86, No. 1, August 31, 2020.

Hidayatullah, Nur Luthfi, "Middle Power's Role in Health Diplomacy During Covid-19: The Case of MIKTA Member States," *Sunan Ampel Review of Political and Social Sciences*, Vol. 1, No. 1, 2021.

Hill, Christopher, and Sarah Beadle, *The Art of Attraction: Soft Power and the UK's Role in the World*, British Academy, 2014.

Hotez, Peter J., "'Vaccine Diplomacy': Historical Perspectives and Future Directions," *PLoS Neglected Tropical Diseases*, Vol. 8, No. 6, 2014.

Jacinto, Leela, "Can the Unmasking of China's Covid-19 'Mask Diplomacy' Stem Beijing's Global Power Grab?" France24, January 5, 2020.

Jeong, Eunsun, Munire Hagose, Hyungul Jung, Moran Ki, and Antoine Flahault, "Understanding South Korea's Response to the COVID-19 Outbreak: A Real-Time Analysis," *International Journal of Environmental Research and Public Health*, Vol. 17, No. 24, December 21, 2020.

Kang, JaHyun, Yun Young Jang, JinHwa Kim, Si-Hyeon Han, Ki Rog Lee, Mukju Kim, and Joong Sik Eom, "South Korea's Responses to Stop the COVID-19 Pandemic," *American Journal of Infection Control*, Vol. 48, No. 9, September 2020.

Katz, Rebecca, Sarah Kornblet, Grace Arnold, Eric Lief, and Julie E. Fischer, "Defining Health Diplomacy: Changing Demands in the Era of Globalization," *Milbank Quarterly*, Vol. 89, No. 3, 2011.

Kickbusch, Ilona, and Austin Liu, "Global Health Diplomacy—Reconstructing Power and Governance," *The Lancet*, 2022.

Kim, Junic, and Kelly Ashihara, "National Disaster Management System: COVID-19 Case in Korea," *International Journal of Environmental Research and Public Health*, Vol. 17, No. 18, September 14, 2020.

Kim, Ji Eon, Ji Ho L Lee, Hocheol Lee, Seok Jun Moon, and Eun Woo Nam, "COVID-19 Screening Center Models in South Korea," *Journal of Public Health Policy*, Vol. 42, No. 1, October 2021.

Lee, Daejoong Kyungmoo Heo, Yongseok Seo, Hyerim Ahn, Kyungran Jung, Sohyun Lee, and Hyeseung Choi, "Flattening the Curve on COVID-19: South Korea's Measures in Tackling Initial Outbreak of Coronavirus," *American Journal of Epidemiology*, Vol. 190, No. 4, April 6, 2021.

Lee, Sang M., and DonHee Lee, "Lessons Learned from Battling COVID-19: The Korean Experience," *International Journal of Environmental Research and Public Health*, Vol. 17, No. 20, October 16, 2020.

Lee, Seow Ting, and Hun Shik Kim, "Nation Branding in the COVID-19 Era: South Korea's Pandemic Public Diplomacy," *Place Branding and Public Diplomacy*, Vol. 17, No. 4, 2021.

Lim, So Hyung, and Kristin Sziarto, "When the Illiberal and the Neoliberal Meet Around Infectious Diseases: An Examination of the MERS Response in South Korea," *Territory, Politics, Governance*, Vol. 8, No. 1, 2020.

Ling, Gabriel Hoh Teck Ling, Nur Amiera Binti Md Suhud, Pau Chung Leng, Lee Bak Yeo, Chin Tiong Cheng, Mohd Hamdan Haji Ahmad, and Ak Mohd Rafiq Ak Matusin, "Factors Influencing Asia-Pacific Countries' Success Level in Curbing COVID-19: A Review Using a Social-Ecological System (SES) Framework," *International Journal of Environmental Research and Public Health*, Vol. 18, No. 4, February 10, 2021.

Martiniuk, Alexandra L. C., Mitra Manouchehrian, Joel A. Negin, and Anthony B. Zwi, "Brain Gains: A Literature Review of Medical Missions to Low and Middle-Income Countries," *BMC Health Services Research*, Vol. 12, No. 1, 2012.

McClory, Jonathan, *The Soft Power 30: A Global Ranking of Soft Power*, Portland PR Limited, 2015.

McClory, Jonathan, *Soft Power 30: A Global Ranking of Soft Power 2019*, Portland PR Limited, 2019.

McClory, Jonathan, *Socially Distanced Diplomacy: The Future of Soft Power and Public Diplomacy in a Fragile World*, Sanctuary Counsel and USC Center on Public Diplomacy, May 2021.

McGinnis, Michael D., and Elinor Ostrom, "Social-Ecological System Framework: Initial Changes and Continuing Challenges," *Ecology and Society*, Vol. 19, No. 2, 2014.

Monocle, "Soft Power Survey 2017/18," video, December 28, 2017. As of August 2, 2022: https://monocle.com/film/affairs/soft-power-survey-2017-18/

Moore, Melinda, Bill Gelfeld, Adeyemi Okunogbe, and Christopher Paul, "Identifying Future Disease Hot Spots: Infectious Disease Vulnerability Index," *RAND Health Quarterly*, Vol. 6, No. 3, 2017. As of July 26, 2022: https://www.rand.org/pubs/periodicals/health-quarterly/issues/v6/n3/05.html

Moradi, Hazhir, and Atefeh Vaezi, "Lessons Learned from Korea: COVID-19 Pandemic," *Infection Control & Hospital Epidemiology*, Vol. 41, No. 7, 2020.

Nye, Joseph S., *Soft Power: The Means to Success in World Politics*, PublicAffairs, 2004.

Nye, Joseph, Soft Power: The Origins and Political Progress of a Concept," Palgrave Communications, Vol. 3, No. 17008, February 2017.

Nye, Joseph S., "Soft Power and Public Diplomacy Revisited," in "Debating Public Diplomacy: Now and Next," special issue, *Hague Journal of Diplomacy*, Vol. 14, Nos. 1–2, April 2019.

Oh, Juhwan, Jong-Koo Lee, Dan Schwarz, Hannah L. Ratcliffe, Jeffrey F. Markuns, and Lisa R. Hirschhorn, "National Response to COVID-19 in the Republic of Korea and Lessons Learned for Other Countries," *Health Systems & Reform, Vol.* 6, No. 1, 2020.

Park, Yoojin, In Sil Huh, Jaekyung Lee, Cho Ryok Kang, Sung il Cho, Hyon Jeen Ham, Hea Sook Kim, Jung il Kim, Baeg Ju Na, and Jin Yong Lee, "Application of Testing-Tracing-Treatment Strategy in Response to the COVID-19 Outbreak in Seoul, Korea," *Journal of Korean Medical Science*, Vol. 35, No. 45, November 23, 2020.

Rokni, Ladan, and Sam-Hun Park, "Measures to Control the Transmission of COVID-19 in South Korea: Searching for the Hidden Effective Factors," *Asia Pacific Journal of Public Health*, Vol. 32, No. 8, 2020.

Schaller, Bettina "What the Rest of the World Can Learn from South Korea's COVID-19 Response," webpage, December 15, 2020. As of July 26, 2022: https://www.adeccogroup.com/future-of-work/latest-insights/what-the-rest-of-the-world-can-learn-from-south-korea/

Shakeel, Shahella Idrees, Matthew Brown, Shakeel Sethi, and Tim K Mackey, "Achieving the End Game: Employing "Vaccine Diplomacy" to Eradicate Polio in Pakistan," *BMC Public Health*, Vol. 19, No. 1, 2019.

Shuren, Jeffrey, and Timothy Stenzel, "South Korea's Implementation of a COVID-19 National Testing Strategy," *Health Affairs*, May 25, 2021.

Suhud, Nur Amiera, Gabriel Hoh Teck Ling, Pau Chung Leng, and A. K. Muhamad Rafiq A. K. Matusin, "Using A Socio-Ecological System (SES) Framework to Explain Factors Influencing Countries' Success Level in Curbing COVID-19," webpage, medRxiv, 2020.

Soft Power 30, "Overall Ranking 2019," homepage, 2019. https://softpower30.com/

Soft Power 30, "South Korea: 2019 Overview," webpage, 2015–2019. As of July 26, 2022: https://softpower30.com/country/south-korea/

SP30—*See* Soft Power 30.

Verma, Raj, "China's 'Mask Diplomacy' to Change the COVID-19 Narrative in Europe," *Asia Europe Journal*, Vol. 18, No. 2, 2020.

Watkins, Meredith, "Health Diplomacy: Soft Power to Battle Global Threats," Duke University Center for International and Global Studies, March 30, 2020.

WHO—*See* World Health Organization.

"Why Korea Rushed to Raise Coronavirus Threat Level to Highest," *Korea Biomedical Review*, February 2020.

World Health Organization, *Joint External Evaluation of IHR Core Capacities of the United States of America,* mission report, June 2016.

World Health Organization, *Joint External Evaluation of IHR Core Capacities of the Republic of Korea,* mission report, 28 August–1 September 2017, 2017a.

World Health Organization, *Joint External Evaluation of IHR Core Capacities of the Republic of Indonesia*, mission report, 20–24 November 2017b.

World Health Organization, *Joint External Evaluation Tool: International Health Regulations (2005)*, 2nd ed., 2018.

Yang, Yuseon, Hyejung Kim, and Jieun Hwang, "Quarantine Facility for Patients with COVID-19 with Mild Symptoms in Korea: Experience from Eighteen Residential Treatment Centers," *Journal of Korean Medical Science*, Vol. 35, No. 49, December 21, 2020.

Zeng, Kylie, Stephanie N. Bernardo, and Weldon E. Havins, "The Use of Digital Tools to Mitigate the COVID-19 Pandemic: Comparative Retrospective Study of Six Countries," *JMIR Public Health and Surveillance*, Vol. 6, No. 4, December 23, 2020.

Zhu, Zhongming, and Wei Liu, *Assessment of COVID-19 Response in the Republic of Korea*, Asia Development Bank, 2021.